The

Seven-Day

Gallbladder

Diet Plan

Jerry V. Hatcher

Table of Contents

Introduction

In the intricate symphony of human physiology, the gallbladder plays a vital role as a small yet indispensable instrument. Nestled beneath the liver, this pear-shaped organ undertakes the task of storing bile—nature's emulsifier—until it's summoned to aid in the digestion of fats. Just as a finely tuned instrument requires care to perform at its best, so does the gallbladder demand attention and mindful nourishment to maintain its health and functionality.

The Gallbladder Diet, a nuanced and purposeful culinary approach, emerges as a guiding light for those seeking to cultivate balance and well-being within their digestive system. This dietary strategy emphasizes the consumption of foods that are gentle on the gallbladder, reducing the risk of gallstones and promoting optimal digestion. Rich in whole grains, lean proteins, fresh fruits, and vegetables, this diet finds its strength in a harmonious blend of nutrients that honor both taste and health.

Navigating the realms of gastronomy, this diet becomes an exploration of flavors, textures, and ingredients that not only invigorate the palate but also fortify the body. From the robust savoriness of Baked Salmon with Lemon and Dill to the delicate balance of Spinach and Feta Stuffed Chicken Breast, each dish showcases the potential for culinary excellence while nurturing the gallbladder's needs.

This diet is more than just a collection of recipes; it's an invitation to embark on a journey of self-care and mindful nourishment. By choosing nutrient-dense, gallbladder-friendly ingredients, you empower yourself to embrace a lifestyle that fosters vitality and digestive wellness. Throughout this guide, you'll discover a diverse array of delectable creations, from comforting soups to vibrant salads and enticing entrees, all thoughtfully designed to support your gallbladder's health.

Join us as we delve into a seven-day exploration of flavors and nourishment, celebrating the gallbladder's unique role in our well-being. From tantalizing your taste buds to embracing the wisdom of holistic health, the Gallbladder Diet invites you to experience the harmonious union of mindful eating and culinary delight. Let us embark on this journey together,

honoring our bodies and savoring each delicious
moment along the way.

<h1 style="text-align:center"><u>Chapter 1</u></h1>

<u>Wholesome Recipes for Gallbladder Wellness</u>

1. Baked Salmon with Lemon and Dill: A heart-healthy and delicious option, this baked salmon is seasoned with the bright flavors of lemon and aromatic dill, providing essential omega-3 fatty acids and a burst of refreshing taste.

- Ingredients:

    - 4 salmon fillets

    - 2 tablespoons fresh lemon juice

    - 2 teaspoons fresh dill, chopped

    - 2 tablespoons olive oil

    - Salt and pepper to taste

  - Instructions:

    1. Preheat the oven to 375°F (190°C). Place the salmon fillets on a baking sheet lined with parchment paper.

4

2. In a small bowl, mix the lemon juice, dill, olive oil, salt, and pepper.

3. Brush the lemon-dill mixture over the salmon fillets, ensuring they are evenly coated.

4. Bake the salmon in the preheated oven for about 15-20 minutes or until the salmon is cooked through and flakes easily with a fork.

5. Serve the baked salmon with your choice of side dishes and enjoy!

2. Quinoa and Roasted Vegetable Salad: A nutrient-rich and satisfying salad featuring protein-packed quinoa and a medley of roasted vegetables, tossed in a light dressing for a delightful combination of flavors and textures.

- Ingredients:

    - 1 cup quinoa, rinsed

    - 2 cups mixed vegetables (e.g., bell peppers, zucchini, cherry tomatoes)

    - 2 tablespoons olive oil

    - 1 teaspoon dried oregano

- Salt and pepper to taste

- 2 tablespoons fresh lemon juice

- 1/4 cup fresh parsley, chopped

- Instructions:

1. Preheat the oven to 400°F (200°C). Toss the mixed vegetables with olive oil, dried oregano, salt, and pepper.

2. Spread the seasoned vegetables on a baking sheet and roast for about 20-25 minutes, or until they are tender and slightly charred.

3. In the meantime, cook the quinoa according to the package instructions.

4. Once the quinoa and roasted vegetables are ready, combine them in a large bowl. Drizzle with fresh lemon juice and toss in chopped parsley.

5. Adjust seasoning as needed, and the quinoa and roasted vegetable salad is ready to be served warm or chilled!

3. Steamed Broccoli with a Sprinkle of Lemon Zest:
Simple yet nutritious, steamed broccoli is enhanced

with a touch of fresh lemon zest, delivering vital nutrients and a zesty twist to this green favorite.

- Ingredients:

    - 2 cups broccoli florets

    - Zest of 1 lemon

    - 1 tablespoon olive oil

    - Salt and pepper to taste

  - Instructions:

    1. Steam the broccoli florets until they are tender-crisp. You can use a steamer basket or microwave for this step.

    2. In a serving bowl, drizzle the steamed broccoli with olive oil and gently toss to coat.

    3. Sprinkle the lemon zest over the broccoli and season with salt and pepper to taste.

    4. Serve immediately as a nutritious and refreshing side dish.

4. Grilled Chicken Breast with Rosemary: Tender and lean grilled chicken breast infused with the delightful aroma of rosemary, offering a protein-rich and savory dish.

- Ingredients:

    - 4 boneless, skinless chicken breasts

    - 2 tablespoons olive oil

    - 2 cloves garlic, minced

    - 1 tablespoon fresh rosemary, chopped

    - Salt and pepper to taste

- Instructions:

    1. Preheat the grill or grill pan over medium-high heat.

    2. In a bowl, combine olive oil, minced garlic, chopped rosemary, salt, and pepper.

    3. Brush both sides of the chicken breasts with the olive oil mixture.

    4. Grill the chicken breasts for approximately 6-7 minutes per side or until they are fully cooked and have grill marks.

5. Remove from the grill, let them rest for a few minutes, and then serve with your favorite sides.

5. Lentil Soup with Carrots and Spinach: A comforting and hearty soup, this lentil-based creation is combined with vibrant carrots and nutrient-dense spinach, providing a warm and nourishing meal.

- Ingredients:

  - 1 cup dried green or red lentils, rinsed

  - 1 tablespoon olive oil

  - 1 onion, chopped

  - 2 cloves garlic, minced

  - 2 carrots, diced

  - 4 cups vegetable or chicken broth

  - 1 cup fresh spinach, chopped

  - 1 teaspoon dried thyme

  - Salt and pepper to taste

- Instructions:

1. In a large pot, heat olive oil over medium heat. Add chopped onions and sauté until they become translucent.

2. Stir in minced garlic and diced carrots, and cook for an additional 2-3 minutes.

3. Add the rinsed lentils, vegetable or chicken broth, and dried thyme to the pot. Bring to a boil, then reduce heat to a simmer and cover the pot.

4. Let the lentil soup simmer for about 20-25 minutes or until the lentils are tender.

5. Stir in the chopped spinach and season with salt and pepper to taste. Simmer for a few more minutes until the spinach wilts.

6. Serve the comforting lentil soup hot and enjoy the wholesome flavors.

6. Grilled Zucchini and Squash Medley: Colorful zucchini and squash, grilled to perfection with selected seasonings, create a light and tasty side dish rich in vitamins and minerals.

- Ingredients:

- 2 zucchinis, sliced

- 2 yellow squashes, sliced

- 2 tablespoons olive oil

- 1 teaspoon dried Italian herbs (oregano, basil, thyme)

- Salt and pepper to taste

- Instructions:

1. Preheat the grill or grill pan over medium-high heat.

2. In a bowl, toss the zucchini and squash slices with olive oil, dried Italian herbs, salt, and pepper.

3. Grill the zucchini and squash slices for about 3-4 minutes per side or until they have grill marks and are tender.

4. Transfer the grilled vegetables to a serving platter and serve as a delightful side dish.

7. Baked Sweet Potato Fries: A healthier alternative to traditional fries, these baked sweet potato fries are crispy, flavorful, and packed with fiber and essential nutrients.

- Ingredients:

    - 2 large sweet potatoes, cut into fries

    - 2 tablespoons olive oil

    - 1 teaspoon paprika

    - 1/2 teaspoon garlic powder

    - Salt and pepper to taste

- Instructions:

1. Preheat the oven to 425°F (220°C) and line a baking sheet with parchment paper.

2. In a bowl, toss the sweet potato fries with olive oil, paprika, garlic powder, salt, and pepper until evenly coated.

3. Spread the seasoned sweet potato fries in a single layer on the prepared baking sheet.

4. Bake in the preheated oven for about 20-25 minutes, flipping halfway through, until the fries are crispy and golden brown.

5. Remove from the oven, let them cool slightly, and serve as a healthier alternative to traditional fries.

8. Brown Rice and Black Bean Burrito Bowl: A wholesome and balanced bowl, featuring brown rice, protein-rich black beans, and a variety of fresh toppings for a delicious and satisfying meal.

- Ingredients:

    - 1 cup cooked brown rice

    - 1 cup black beans (canned or cooked)

    - 1 cup cherry tomatoes, halved

    - 1 avocado, diced

    - 1/4 cup red onion, finely chopped

    - 2 tablespoons fresh cilantro, chopped

    - Juice of 1 lime

    - Salt and pepper to taste

- Instructions:

    1. In a bowl, combine cooked brown rice, black beans, cherry tomatoes, diced avocado, chopped red onion, and fresh cilantro.

    2. Squeeze lime juice over the mixture and toss everything together gently.

    3. Season with salt and pepper to taste.

4. Serve the delicious burrito bowl as is or add your favorite toppings like salsa or Greek yogurt.

9. Poached Eggs over Steamed Asparagus: A delightful breakfast choice, poached eggs served atop tender steamed asparagus, providing a protein-packed and nourishing start to the day.

  - Ingredients:

    - 4 large eggs

    - 1 bunch asparagus spears, trimmed

    - 1 tablespoon white vinegar

    - Salt and pepper to taste

  - Instructions:

    1. Fill a large pot with water and bring it to a gentle simmer. Add the white vinegar to the water.

    2. Carefully crack each egg into a small cup or ramekin.

3. Place the trimmed asparagus spears into a steamer basket and steam until tender-crisp.

4. Create a gentle whirlpool in the simmering water and slide one egg into the center. Repeat with the other eggs.

5. Poach the eggs for about 3-4 minutes or until the whites are set but the yolks are still runny.

6. Remove the poached eggs with a slotted spoon and drain any excess water.

7. Arrange the steamed asparagus on a plate and top with the poached eggs. Season with salt and pepper to taste.

10. Turkey and Vegetable Stir-Fry: A quick and nutritious stir-fry featuring lean turkey and an assortment of colorful vegetables, seasoned with aromatic herbs and spices for a flavorful dish.

 - Ingredients:

   - 1 lb. (450g) lean turkey breast, thinly sliced

   - 2 cups broccoli florets

   - 1 red bell pepper, sliced

- 1 yellow bell pepper, sliced

- 1 tablespoon ginger, minced

- 2 cloves garlic, minced

- 2 tablespoons low-sodium soy sauce

- 1 tablespoon hoisin sauce (optional for added flavor)

- 2 tablespoons olive oil

- Salt and pepper to taste

- Instructions:

1. In a large skillet or wok, heat olive oil over medium-high heat.

2. Add the sliced turkey to the skillet and stir-fry until it is cooked through and lightly browned. Season with salt and pepper.

3. Remove the turkey from the skillet and set it aside.

4. In the same skillet, add a little more oil if needed and stir-fry the minced ginger and garlic until fragrant.

5. Add the broccoli and bell peppers to the skillet, and stir-fry for a few minutes until they are tender-crisp.

6. Return the cooked turkey to the skillet, and add low-sodium soy sauce and hoisin sauce (if using).

7. Toss everything together until the sauce coats the turkey and vegetables evenly.

8. Serve the flavorful turkey and vegetable stir-fry over brown rice or quinoa for a wholesome and satisfying meal.

11. Greek Yogurt with Fresh Berries and a Drizzle of Honey:

- Ingredients:

    - 1 cup Greek yogurt

    - 1/2 cup fresh berries (blueberries, strawberries, raspberries)

    - 1 tablespoon honey

  - Instructions:

    1. In a bowl, spoon the Greek yogurt.

    2. Top the yogurt with the fresh berries.

    3. Drizzle honey over the yogurt and berries.

4. Enjoy this delicious and nutritious Greek yogurt parfait for breakfast or a satisfying snack.

12. Spinach and Feta Stuffed Chicken Breast:

Juicy chicken breast stuffed with a flavorful mix of spinach and tangy feta cheese, creating a savory and wholesome entrée that is sure to impress with its burst of Mediterranean-inspired flavors.

  - Ingredients:

    - 4 boneless, skinless chicken breasts

    - 2 cups fresh spinach, chopped

    - 1/2 cup crumbled feta cheese

    - 1 tablespoon olive oil

    - Salt and pepper to taste

  - Instructions:

    1. Preheat the oven to 375°F (190°C).

    2. Cut a slit horizontally through the thickest part of each chicken breast to create a pocket without cutting through the other side.

3. Season the inside of the chicken breasts with salt and pepper.

4. Stuff each chicken breast with chopped spinach and crumbled feta cheese, pressing the filling firmly.

5. Heat olive oil in an oven-safe skillet over medium-high heat. Sear the stuffed chicken breasts for 2-3 minutes per side until golden brown.

6. Transfer the skillet to the preheated oven and bake for about 15-20 minutes or until the chicken is cooked through and the cheese is melted.

7. Remove from the oven, let the chicken rest for a few minutes, and serve this delightful spinach and feta stuffed chicken breast.

13. Cauliflower Rice with Sautéed Mushrooms and Garlic:

A low-carb alternative to traditional rice, cauliflower rice is sautéed with earthy mushrooms and aromatic garlic, resulting in a tasty and satisfying side dish suitable for various dietary preferences.

 - Ingredients:

  - 1 medium cauliflower head, grated into rice-like texture

- 1 cup mushrooms, sliced

- 2 cloves garlic, minced

- 2 tablespoons olive oil

- Salt and pepper to taste

- Instructions:

1. Heat olive oil in a large skillet over medium heat.

2. Add minced garlic and sliced mushrooms to the skillet. Sauté until the mushrooms are tender and lightly browned.

3. Add the cauliflower rice to the skillet, and season with salt and pepper to taste.

4. Cook the cauliflower rice and mushrooms, stirring occasionally, for about 5-7 minutes or until the cauliflower is tender and cooked through.

5. Serve this flavorful and low-carb cauliflower rice as a side dish or as a base for your favorite stir-fries or grain bowls.

14. Oven-Roasted Brussels Sprouts with a Dash of Olive Oil:

Nutrient-packed Brussels sprouts roasted to perfection with a light drizzle of olive oil, offering a delectable and nutritious vegetable dish that is both easy to prepare and full of flavor.

- Ingredients:

    - 1 lb (450g) Brussels sprouts, trimmed and halved

    - 2 tablespoons olive oil

    - Salt and pepper to taste

- Instructions:

    1. Preheat the oven to 400°F (200°C).

    2. In a large bowl, toss the halved Brussels sprouts with olive oil, salt, and pepper until evenly coated.

    3. Spread the seasoned Brussels sprouts in a single layer on a baking sheet lined with parchment paper.

    4. Roast in the preheated oven for about 20-25 minutes or until the Brussels sprouts are crispy and lightly charred on the edges.

    5. Remove from the oven and serve these delicious oven-roasted Brussels sprouts as a nutritious and flavorful side dish.

15. Quinoa and Kale Stuffed Peppers:

Colorful bell peppers filled with a hearty mixture of quinoa and nutrient-rich kale, providing a wholesome and balanced meal that is rich in vitamins and plant-based protein.

 - Ingredients:

   - 4 bell peppers (any color), tops cut off and seeds removed

   - 1 cup cooked quinoa

   - 2 cups kale, chopped

   - 1 tablespoon olive oil

   - 1/2 cup feta cheese (optional for extra flavor)

   - Salt and pepper to taste

 - Instructions:

   1. Preheat the oven to 375°F (190°C).

   2. In a large skillet, heat olive oil over medium heat. Sauté the chopped kale until wilted and tender.

   3. In a mixing bowl, combine cooked quinoa, sautéed kale, and feta cheese (if using). Season with salt and pepper to taste.

4. Stuff each bell pepper with the quinoa and kale mixture, pressing it down gently.

5. Place the stuffed peppers in a baking dish and cover it with foil.

6. Bake in the preheated oven for 25-30 minutes or until the peppers are tender.

7. Remove from the oven and let the stuffed peppers cool slightly before serving. Enjoy this vibrant and nutritious quinoa and kale stuffed peppers as a satisfying main course.

16. Turkey Meatballs with Marinara Sauce:

Lean ground turkey meatballs simmered in a savory marinara sauce, creating a delicious and protein-rich addition to pasta, sandwiches, or served as an appetizer.

  - Ingredients:

    - 1 lb (450g) ground turkey

    - 1/2 cup breadcrumbs (gluten-free if needed)

- 1/4 cup grated Parmesan cheese

- 1 large egg

- 2 cloves garlic, minced

- 1 teaspoon dried oregano

- 1 teaspoon dried basil

- Salt and pepper to taste

- 2 cups marinara sauce

- Instructions:

1. Preheat the oven to 375°F (190°C).

2. In a large bowl, combine ground turkey, breadcrumbs, grated Parmesan cheese, egg, minced garlic, dried oregano, dried basil, salt, and pepper. Mix until well combined.

3. Form the mixture into meatballs of desired size and place them on a baking sheet lined with parchment paper.

4. Bake the turkey meatballs in the preheated oven for 15-20 minutes or until cooked through and lightly browned.

5. Warm the marinara sauce in a saucepan over medium heat.

6. Add the baked turkey meatballs to the marinara sauce and simmer for a few minutes until the meatballs are coated with the sauce.

7. Serve the turkey meatballs with marinara sauce over pasta or as an appetizer with toothpicks.

17. Steamed Artichokes with a Lemon-Garlic Dipping Sauce:

Tender artichokes steamed to perfection, served with a zesty lemon-garlic dipping sauce for a delightful and healthy appetizer or side dish that celebrates the unique flavor of artichokes.

- Ingredients:

    - 2 large artichokes

    - 1 lemon, sliced

    - 3 cloves garlic, minced

    - 1/4 cup mayonnaise

    - 2 tablespoons olive oil

    - Salt and pepper to taste

- Instructions:

1. Trim the stem of each artichoke and remove any tough outer leaves. Cut off the top of the artichoke, about 1 inch.

2. Place a steamer basket in a large pot filled with water and bring it to a boil. Add the lemon slices to the water.

3. Place the prepared artichokes in the steamer basket, cover the pot, and steam for 30-40 minutes or until the outer leaves can be easily pulled off.

4. In the meantime, prepare the lemon-garlic dipping sauce by mixing minced garlic, mayonnaise, olive oil, salt, and pepper in a small bowl.

5. Once the artichokes are steamed, remove them from the steamer basket and serve with the lemon-garlic dipping sauce.

18. Cucumber and Tomato Salad with Light Vinaigrette:

A refreshing and colorful salad combining crisp cucumber and juicy tomatoes, dressed in a light vinaigrette with hints of tanginess and freshness, making it a perfect summer accompaniment.

- Ingredients:

- 1 large cucumber, sliced

- 1 cup cherry tomatoes, halved

- 1/4 cup red onion, thinly sliced

- 2 tablespoons fresh parsley, chopped

- 2 tablespoons olive oil

- 1 tablespoon white wine vinegar

- 1 teaspoon Dijon mustard

- Salt and pepper to taste

- Instructions:

1. In a large bowl, combine cucumber slices, halved cherry tomatoes, thinly sliced red onion, and chopped parsley.

2. In a separate small bowl, whisk together olive oil, white wine vinegar, Dijon mustard, salt, and pepper to make the vinaigrette dressing.

3. Pour the vinaigrette over the cucumber and tomato mixture. Toss everything together until well coated.

4. Serve the refreshing cucumber and tomato salad immediately, or refrigerate it for a short time to allow the flavors to meld.

19. Baked Cod with a Herb and Garlic Crust:

Tender cod fillets coated with a flavorful crust made from a blend of aromatic herbs and garlic, resulting in a delicious and nutritious seafood dish that is simple to prepare yet bursting with taste.

- Ingredients:

    - 4 cod fillets

    - 2 tablespoons olive oil

    - 1 tablespoon fresh parsley, chopped

    - 1 tablespoon fresh thyme, chopped

    - 2 cloves garlic, minced

    - 1/4 cup breadcrumbs (gluten-free if needed)

    - Salt and pepper to taste

- Instructions:

    1. Preheat the oven to 400°F (200°C). Grease a baking dish with olive oil or line it with parchment paper.

    2. In a small bowl, mix chopped parsley, chopped thyme, minced garlic, breadcrumbs, salt, and pepper.

3. Brush both sides of the cod fillets with olive oil and place them in the prepared baking dish.

4. Press the herb and garlic mixture on top of each cod fillet, forming a crust.

5. Bake the cod in the preheated oven for about 12-15 minutes or until it is cooked through and easily flakes with a fork.

6. Serve the baked cod with a herb and garlic crust alongside your favorite sides.

20. Grilled Shrimp Skewers with Bell Peppers and Onions:

 - Ingredients:

   - 1 lb (450g) large shrimp, peeled and deveined

   - 1 red bell pepper, cut into chunks

   - 1 yellow bell pepper, cut into chunks

   - 1 red onion, cut into chunks

   - 2 tablespoons olive oil

   - 1 teaspoon smoked paprika

   - 1/2 teaspoon garlic powder

- Salt and pepper to taste

- Wooden or metal skewers

- Instructions:

1. If using wooden skewers, soak them in water for at least 30 minutes to prevent burning during grilling.

2. In a large bowl, toss shrimp, bell pepper chunks, and red onion chunks with olive oil, smoked paprika, garlic powder, salt, and pepper until well coated.

3. Thread the shrimp, bell peppers, and onions onto the skewers alternately.

4. Preheat the grill or grill pan over medium-high heat. Grill the shrimp skewers for about 2-3 minutes per side or until the shrimp are pink and cooked through.

5. Remove the grilled shrimp skewers from the heat and serve them as a flavorful and protein-packed main course or appetizer.

Succulent shrimp skewers paired with colorful bell peppers and onions, grilled to perfection, creating a mouthwatering and protein-packed meal with a delightful blend of textures and flavors.

21. Baked Apple Slices Sprinkled with Cinnamon:

Sliced apples baked to perfection and sprinkled with aromatic cinnamon, creating a warm and comforting dessert that highlights the natural sweetness of the fruit without added sugars.

- Ingredients:

    - 2 large apples, cored and thinly sliced

    - 1 teaspoon ground cinnamon

    - Instructions:

    1. Preheat the oven to 375°F (190°C).

    2. Arrange the apple slices in a single layer on a baking sheet lined with parchment paper.

    3. Sprinkle ground cinnamon over the apple slices.

    4. Bake in the preheated oven for about 15-20 minutes or until the apples are tender and slightly caramelized.

    5. Remove from the oven and let the baked apple slices cool for a few minutes before serving. Enjoy this warm and naturally sweet treat.

22. Tofu and Vegetable Stir-Fry:

A delicious and protein-rich stir-fry featuring tofu and an array of fresh vegetables, stir-fried with a savory sauce for a plant-based meal that is both flavorful and nutritious.

- Ingredients:

    - 1 block (14 oz) firm tofu, drained and cut into cubes

    - 2 cups mixed vegetables (e.g., bell peppers, broccoli, carrots, snap peas)

    - 2 tablespoons soy sauce (or tamari for a gluten-free option)

    - 1 tablespoon hoisin sauce

    - 1 tablespoon sesame oil

    - 2 cloves garlic, minced

    - 1 tablespoon fresh ginger, grated

    - 2 green onions, sliced

    - 1 tablespoon sesame seeds (optional for garnish)

    - Cooked rice or noodles (for serving)

- Instructions:

    1. In a large skillet or wok, heat sesame oil over medium-high heat.

2. Add minced garlic and grated ginger to the skillet and stir-fry for about 30 seconds until fragrant.

3. Add cubed tofu to the skillet and cook until it is lightly browned on all sides.

4. Stir in the mixed vegetables and cook until they are tender-crisp.

5. In a small bowl, mix soy sauce and hoisin sauce, then pour the sauce over the tofu and vegetables. Toss everything together until coated.

6. Garnish the tofu and vegetable stir-fry with sliced green onions and sesame seeds.

7. Serve the flavorful stir-fry over cooked rice or noodles for a satisfying and wholesome plant-based meal.

23. Butternut Squash Soup with a Hint of Nutmeg:

Creamy butternut squash soup seasoned with a subtle hint of nutmeg, delivering a comforting and velvety soup with a rich blend of flavors.

 - Ingredients:

 - 1 medium butternut squash, peeled, seeded, and cut into chunks

 - 1 onion, chopped

- 2 cloves garlic, minced

- 4 cups vegetable or chicken broth

- 1/2 cup coconut milk (or heavy cream for a richer version)

- 1/4 teaspoon ground nutmeg

- Salt and pepper to taste

- Fresh parsley or chives (for garnish)

- Instructions:

1. In a large pot, sauté chopped onion and minced garlic until the onion becomes translucent.

2. Add the butternut squash chunks and vegetable or chicken broth to the pot. Bring to a boil, then reduce heat and simmer until the squash is tender.

3. Using an immersion blender or a regular blender, puree the soup until smooth and creamy.

4. Stir in coconut milk (or heavy cream) and ground nutmeg. Season with salt and pepper to taste.

5. Reheat the soup if necessary before serving.

6. Garnish each bowl of butternut squash soup with fresh parsley or chives.

7. Enjoy the comforting and flavorful butternut squash soup on its own or with a slice of crusty bread.

24. Shredded Chicken and Avocado Lettuce Wraps:

Tender shredded chicken and creamy avocado wrapped in crisp lettuce leaves, providing a light and refreshing meal option that is packed with protein and healthy fats.

- Ingredients:

  - 2 cups cooked and shredded chicken breast

  - 2 ripe avocados, peeled and diced

  - 1/4 cup red onion, finely chopped

  - 1/4 cup cherry tomatoes, halved

  - 2 tablespoons fresh cilantro, chopped

  - 1 tablespoon lime juice

  - Salt and pepper to taste

  - Lettuce leaves (such as romaine or butter lettuce)

- Instructions:

1. In a large bowl, combine shredded chicken, diced avocado, chopped red onion, halved cherry tomatoes, and chopped cilantro.

2. Drizzle lime juice over the mixture and gently toss everything together.

3. Season with salt and pepper to taste.

4. Spoon the chicken and avocado mixture into individual lettuce leaves, creating lettuce wraps.

5. Serve these refreshing and protein-packed lettuce wraps as a light lunch or appetizer.

25. Baked Pears with a Drizzle of Honey and a Sprinkle of Cinnamon:

Ripe pears baked until tender, then drizzled with honey and dusted with cinnamon for a naturally sweet and wholesome dessert that is both delightful and easy to prepare.

 - Ingredients:

   - 4 ripe pears, halved and cored

   - 2 tablespoons honey

- 1/2 teaspoon ground cinnamon

- Instructions:

1. Preheat the oven to 375°F (190°C).

2. Place the pear halves on a baking sheet lined with parchment paper, cut side up.

3. Drizzle honey over each pear half and sprinkle ground cinnamon on top.

4. Bake in the preheated oven for about 20-25 minutes or until the pears are tender and slightly caramelized.

5. Remove from the oven and let the baked pears cool for a few minutes.

6. Serve the warm and naturally sweet baked pears as a delicious and healthy dessert. You can also add a dollop of Greek yogurt or a sprinkle of chopped nuts for added texture and flavor. Enjoy!

Chapter 2

Seven day meal plan

Here's a sample seven-day meal plan featuring the twenty-five recipes for the gallbladder diet:

Day 1:

- Breakfast: Greek Yogurt with Fresh Berries and a Drizzle of Honey

- Lunch: Lentil Soup with Carrots and Spinach

- Dinner: Baked Salmon with Lemon and Dill, served with Steamed Broccoli with a Sprinkle of Lemon Zest

Day 2:

- Breakfast: Quinoa and Kale Stuffed Peppers

- Lunch: Turkey and Vegetable Stir-Fry

- Dinner: Butternut Squash Soup with a Hint of Nutmeg, served with Baked Cod with a Herb and Garlic Crust

Day 3:

- Breakfast: Baked Apple Slices Sprinkled with Cinnamon

- Lunch: Tofu and Vegetable Stir-Fry

- Dinner: Grilled Chicken Breast with Rosemary, served with Grilled Zucchini and Squash Medley

Day 4:

- Breakfast: Greek Yogurt with Fresh Berries and a Drizzle of Honey

- Lunch: Spinach and Feta Stuffed Chicken Breast, served with Quinoa and Roasted Vegetable Salad

- Dinner: Cauliflower Rice with Sautéed Mushrooms and Garlic

Day 5:

- Breakfast: Poached Eggs over Steamed Asparagus

- Lunch: Turkey Meatballs with Marinara Sauce, served with Oven-Roasted Brussels Sprouts with a Dash of Olive Oil

- Dinner: Baked Sweet Potato Fries, served with Shredded Chicken and Avocado Lettuce Wraps

Day 6:

- Breakfast: Baked Pears with a Drizzle of Honey and a Sprinkle of Cinnamon

- Lunch: Quinoa and Kale Stuffed Peppers

- Dinner: Steamed Artichokes with a Lemon-Garlic Dipping Sauce, served with Grilled Shrimp Skewers with Bell Peppers and Onions

Day 7:

- Breakfast: Greek Yogurt with Fresh Berries and a Drizzle of Honey

- Lunch: Baked Cod with a Herb and Garlic Crust, served with Steamed Broccoli with a Sprinkle of Lemon Zest

- Dinner: Butternut Squash Soup with a Hint of Nutmeg, served with Tofu and Vegetable Stir-Fry

This is just a sample, so remember that you can adjust these meals according to your preferences.

Conclusion

Embarking on this 7-day gallbladder diet journey promises not only a symphony of flavors but also a harmonious dance between wholesome nutrition and culinary delight. From the zesty embrace of Baked Salmon with Lemon and Dill to the comforting warmth of Butternut Squash Soup with a Hint of Nutmeg, each plate tells a tale of nourishment and well-being.

This carefully curated meal plan presents an array of dishes that cater to both your taste buds and your gallbladder's needs. We've embraced the vibrant colors of nature with Quinoa and Kale Stuffed Peppers, celebrated the succulence of lean proteins with Turkey Meatballs in Marinara Sauce, and indulged in the sweetness of Baked Pears drizzled with honey and a sprinkle of cinnamon.

As you savor the interplay of textures and aromas, remember that this journey isn't just about the meals—

it's a celebration of mindful eating, where the nourishment of body and soul comes together in every bite. Whether you're sipping on nutrient-rich Lentil Soup or crafting an artful blend of Tofu and Vegetable Stir-Fry, you're making a conscious choice to honor your well-being.

So, as you embark on this culinary adventure, let the flavors ignite your senses and the carefully selected ingredients guide your path to a healthier you. May these seven days be a testament to the joy of eating well, and a reminder that nourishing your body is a journey worth savoring.

About the author

Jerry V. Hatcher is a culinary virtuoso and the creative mind behind a collection of exquisite cookbooks that transcend the ordinary. With a passion for gastronomy and a flair for culinary artistry, Jerry has crafted a series of cookbooks that take readers on a delectable journey through the world of flavors.

Through his cookbooks, Jerry V. Hatcher combines the finest ingredients with meticulous instructions, ensuring every recipe is a delightful masterpiece waiting to be savored. From tantalizing appetizers to mouthwatering main courses and divine desserts, each page is a celebration of culinary excellence.

With a keen eye for detail, Jerry's cookbooks go beyond the recipes, providing valuable tips, techniques, and personal insights that elevate the cooking experience to new heights. Whether you're a seasoned chef or a culinary enthusiast exploring the kitchen for the first time, Jerry's books cater to all skill levels, fostering confidence and creativity in every home cook.

Each recipe in Jerry V. Hatcher's cookbooks is a reflection of his commitment to authenticity and a passion for diverse cuisines. Drawing inspiration from global flavors and local delicacies, Jerry's culinary creations celebrate the richness of cultures and the joy of sharing food with loved ones. Indulge your passion for cooking and elevate your culinary skills with the culinary masterpieces crafted by Jerry V. Hatcher. Get ready to embark on a gastronomic adventure that will leave you hungry for more, one delicious recipe at a time.

<u>My Little Request</u>

If you have gotten to this point, chances are high you have finished this book.

Thank You for Reading My Book!

I love hearing what you have to say.

I need your input to make the next version of this

book and my future books better.

Please take two minutes now to leave a helpful review on Amazon letting me know what you thought of the book

Thanks so much!

- Jerry V. Hatcher

* 9 7 9 8 8 5 6 1 0 7 8 2 0 *